–I'M NOT YOUR–
SUPERWOMAN

—I'M NOT YOUR—
SUPERWOMAN

LESSONS LEARNED IN RESILIENCY FROM A CAREGIVER'S PERSPECTIVE

PIPPA MAHA

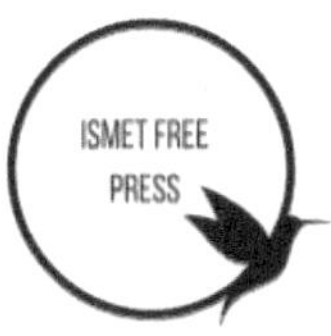
ISMET FREE
PRESS

DEDICATION

To my children, Yakoub, Amaka, and Saraya.

To all the caregivers out there who are finding their balance.

TABLE OF CONTENTS

FOREWORD

Philippa Maha, the mother of 3 children, cares for her youngest child, struggling with the daily uncertainty and maladies of sickle cell. Philippa has worked hard to manage and balance her everyday life, career, and the extraordinary medical needs of her youngest child. She shares her lifelong experience, feelings, and emotions to offer hope to other parents with children with unique medical needs. Sickle cell is just one of many chronic medical problems that affect families. This book is not just for parents of sickle cell children but offers personal insights and experiences that will resonate with caregivers of children with other chronic medical conditions e.g: autism and juvenile diabetes.

As a Medical Social Worker with 40 years of experience working with families in crisis, ten years working in Adult Protective Services, and 30 years in Medical Social Work and Case Management, I'm Not Your Superwoman offers a personal account that reinforces there are others with similar life experiences. Families often struggle to cope with the medical issues affecting their child's health and family dynamics. I encourage you to take the time to read I'm Not Your Superwoman. You're not alone!

-Daryl Morgan, LMSW Medical Social Worker

PREFACE

I'm Not your Superwoman is exactly what it states and couldn't be far from the truth. Most people who know me would disagree with the statement. I'd always been referred to as a superwoman, but no one knew how fragile I was or how much I was suffering within. I kept my composure, even in the direst circumstances. It was not until a few years ago when the pandemic hit that I sought the courage to tell my story.

I chose to write this book because I wanted to document my experience caring for my daughter who has sickle cell disease. In my book, I try to bring awareness to the disease and how it affects families and caregivers, especially single parents. It relates to the emotional toll on caregivers and loved ones. My daughter, Saraya, is my motivation and inspiration for this book. I am inspired by her resilience and strength as she fights this 'beast.' I have watched her grow and evolve into a strong-willed young teenager and look forward to seeing her flourish into a beautiful young woman.Being a caregiver for a child with sickle cell disease can be a challenging but rewarding experience. Sickle cell disease is a genetic condition that affects the shape of red blood cells, causing them to become rigid and sickle-shaped instead of round. This can lead to pain, fatigue, and other complications. As a caregiver, it is important to understand the disease and its effects on the child, as well as how to provide the best possible care and support.

In writing this book, I have tried to draw inferences and situations that have greatly affected me over the years. I see these not only as obstacles or challenges but also building blocks to me becoming who I am today.

I also draw from the strength of other caregivers who have come before me. Many have had to go through countless trials for their loved ones so that others around the world could benefit from the research. We should not forget those who had to suffer for us to understand and enjoy the results of scientific breakthroughs.

I want to celebrate caregivers the world over, so while this may be specific to my experience with sickle cell anemia, I also wish to remember those who care for loved ones suffering from other life-threatening and life-altering illnesses.

PREFACE

It takes courage and strength to smile even when you know that the prognosis is undesirable. Through this memoir, I hope to inspire other caregivers to be their best selves. I want this book to be used as a tool for caregivers to take control of their own lives and well-being. Although being there for our loved ones is important, maintaining our own mental and emotional health is equally important.

-Pippa Maha
Mother, Caregiver, & Holistic Life Coach
Not Your Superwoman

THERE ARE NO COINCIDENCES

CHAPTER 1

Saraya's birth was kind of perturbing in the sense that she weighed the most out of all of my three kids. She was the last to be born, and I was worried because she was so heavy. I didn't think I had the strength to push her out naturally, but God willing, I did. To me, she came into this world healthy and strong. I had all three of my kids naturally. My first child, Yacoub, was 9 pounds, 8 ounces. My second, Amaka, was 9 pounds, 12 ounces. Then Saraya came in at 10 pounds, 11 ounces. During my pregnancy, I felt heavy, even in a sense outside of the weight I was carrying from my beautiful child that was to be born. Both physically and emotionally. I would look at myself and I would think, "oh my goodness. Am I sure I can push her out!?" Sometimes you think you're not capable of doing the impossible, but I did it.

I found out that Saraya had a cleft palate, but I didn't think much of it. I was a little surprised because I knew no one on either my side or my husband's side of the family that had a birth defect. To me, I felt as if it was just one of those "one in a million" types of things. Quite honestly, I thought to myself, "I wonder if this is because I was stressed out during and just before giving birth to her?"

My pregnancy with Saraya was the most trying. When I say "trying," I mean that the combination of incidents leading up to her birth was difficult. My husband and I were constantly arguing towards the latter end of my pregnancy. It stemmed from issues that he was having with insecurity about being out of work before we conceived our daughter. He was having a tough time, and the stress spilled over to me and our happy home. Wait a minute… this would seem as if I'm making excuses for him, as we women often do. Though I do understand how stressful it can be as a husband being jobless and unable to provide for your family financially, it was even harder being a pregnant wife who worked a fulltime job and endured grief caused by an ornery husband every day.

It wasn't a long birth experience. I carried all my babies to full term. I've always gone full term and a little bit over, so it was the same for Saraya. Sometimes you are calm when you're pregnant; my other pregnancies were easy. This pregnancy was different. I was mentally stressed and extremely emotional.

My contractions started at about 2 am on that March morning. Twelve hours later Saraya was born. Several hours after that, it was like a bittersweet "aha moment," finding out she had sickle cell. I thought to myself, "Oops!" I'd forgotten that when my other children were born, we were told they had the trait.

> ## FACT:
>
> According to the CDC, "if both parents have sickle cell trait, there is a 1 in 2 chance that any child of theirs also will have SCT, if the child inherits the sickle cell gene from one of the parents. Such children will not have symptoms of sickle cell disease, but they can pass SCT on to their children. If both parents have sickle cell trait, there is a 1 in 4 chance that any child of theirs will have sickle cell disease. There is the same 1 in 4 chance that the child will not have SCD or SCT."

ACCEPTING THE TRUTH

When we got the news that she had full sickle cell, at first, I wanted to contest it because I knew that to have full sickle cell, both parents had to have the trait. I was aware that her dad had the trait, but I was not certain about my status. The doctor advised it was important I get tested so they could determine what type of sickle cell she had. The results came back that I have the sickle cell trait. That was something I hadn't anticipated.

They then checked her DNA and determined she has Sickle Beta-Zero Thalassemia. Knowing what type of sickle cell she had would help us move forward with her treatment.

Complications of Beta Thal include delayed growth, bone problems, liver and gallbladder problems, enlarged spleen, enlarged kidneys, diabetes, hypothyroidism, heart problems, and acute chest syndrome. I'll delve into that much later. It all has much to do with genes. If both the parents have traits, then there's always one in four chances that one of the kids will have full sickle cell and the other kids will have the traits. One of the kids may not have anything at all. It's like playing Russian roulette. This was only the beginning of our life with sickle cell.

The medical team sent us a research questionnaire and DNA kit to find out further information on why she had a cleft palate. There were questions about our genealogy, whether or not we had a prior history of the cleft palate, any medication I had taken, my mental status, and my emotional state. While filling out the questionnaire, I lied about my emotional state. It was one of those moments where I wanted to keep my business to myself. When you go through certain things, you don't want everyone to see you in that vulnerable state. I just wanted to focus on the situation at hand with my baby girl without thinking about the stress I had endured prior to her birth.

You see, on the form, there was a question about whether I had felt threatened or stressed out, which I denied. That wasn't even a half-truth though. I was extremely stressed out, but I just marked "no," on the paperwork, as if everything had been good.

SIDENOTE:

Caregivers must be transparent when filling out medical forms and questionnaires because this will allow for a better understanding of the social and economic constraints affecting the caregiver, such as difficulties with transportation to the hospital, not being able to pay for essential bills like utilities or food, and difficulties with finding or keeping jobs due to absenteeism. The medical personnel may be able to better diagnose the issue, understand where you are coming from, and recommend resources that may alleviate your situation.

FROM MARRIAGE VOWS TO MARRIAGE WOWS

My husband and I had been going through a trying time. He'd been out of work for a couple of years, and he was dealing with some insecurities about it to the extent that he would accuse me of being unfaithful while I was at work. As a result, that affected our marriage greatly. We were constantly arguing, even before I got pregnant. Usually, I would stay quiet to avoid escalating the situation, but that would only make matters worse. It got to a point where I had to take a stand for myself by responding. With my pregnancy underway, I just refused to sit back and become complacent.

I remember one particular incident that got bad. It was a couple of weeks before my due date, and I had transitioned to working from home. Rather than going into the office while I was dealing with all of the stress, I didn't want to be at work faking it as if all was well. During this particular argument, he threatened that he was going to break my work laptop. He felt that I was focusing more on my work and that my work was my sustenance. He'd always say that my work was my "power."

He said, "oh, okay, I'll take that power away from you."

I was appalled! It made me upset, but I knew in my mind that something would eventually change for the better. Though at that very moment, I knew my marriage was over.

I wanted to say hurtful things; it took every bit of strength in me not to.

I was pretty upset, and told him, "you know what?! I wouldn't even go down that route with you, because to me, I don't think you are lucid right now. You're not thinking straight."

When he would get into his angry tirades, he would just ramble on. Sometimes people will poke at you to get a reaction, but when you're quiet, they get angry. That's how he was. At the time, I didn't want to argue, but I just had to sit there and stomach it. Pun intended. Get it? That was a play on words, stomach it. Ha ha!

> **SIDENOTE:**
>
> **We have to be very cautious with the things we say because once you make statements that are hurtful to people, even when you apologize, you can't take them back. I was very conscious of this, and that's why I remained silent the majority of times we had arguments.**

He was accustomed to being around people with sickle cell. Quite honestly, I wouldn't say I knew of anyone who was battling with sickle cell. I was aware of the condition, but it was only later on in life that I started to understand its severity. Even growing up as a kid, I know I'd heard of it. Some things you hear just like you hear someone has cancer or any other life-threatening condition. You're aware that they're probably struggling, but it doesn't become real until it happens to you.

I knew he had the trait because he disclosed it to me before we got married. However, I wasn't aware that I had the trait. To the best of my knowledge, no one on my side of the family had it. The topic had never come up.

Back in Nigeria, where I come from before you get married, it's customary to get tested to see if you have the trait. If both partners have the trait, you would be strongly advised of the complications of having kids. If one person has the trait and the other person does not, chances are still that when you have kids, one of your kids will have the trait. The whole idea is for you to know your status, so there are no regrets once you start to build a family.

That's why they stress that before you get married, you should take a sickle cell test. I did not do that. In hindsight, I should have.

I can't stress getting tested enough. It's important, even for those who are adopted. You need to know where you come from, and it opens up a whole discussion. Whether it's your natural family or if you're adopted, things may come up in the medical history that leaves you wondering, "oh, how is that possible? Why is that?"

Your overall health matters, including your mental and physical health. DNA says a lot; it comes from two people. If it's not from your immediate family, like your mother or father, it may be somewhere down the line. I can't stress it enough. It's just so important to know your family's overall health history ahead of being in a similar predicament that my family has experienced. It's always good to know because things don't just happen out of nowhere.

I believe that everything happens for a reason to teach us how to live and respect each other and to be empathetic to what others have experienced. How do we react when faced with life's challenges? I believe we all have an inbuilt survival instinct that kicks in when faced with danger and obstacles. I call it the resilience of the human spirit. It's amazing what we can do with the will and belief to see it through; I guess that's why some people looked at me like a superwoman. What we see or understand as obstacles may well be that silver lining to help us become better individuals. This is how I see my life with sickle cell. I have never for one moment questioned "why me?" or "why my family?" I accept it for what it is. There are no coincidences in life.

REFLECTIONS:

Up to this point, how have you described your caregiving journey? We must practice speaking about our experience in a way that is empowering and not disempowering.

____

____

____

____

____

____

____

____

THE WORLD DOESN'T REVOLVE AROUND...

CHAPTER 2

I was unable to breastfeed Saraya because of her cleft palate. She had difficulty swallowing and needed to have corrective surgery done to close the cleft palate. It was physically and emotionally demanding having to deal with that coupled with knowing she had sickle cell. I'd be remiss if I didn't mention that the doctor explained to me that even though she had sickle cell, she wasn't experiencing any pain at that time because she still had some of my umbilical cord blood in her. The umbilical cord helped to increase her red blood cell count.

However, the older she got, her body would need to make enough red blood cells on its own because eventually, the sickling effect of the red blood cells would lead to a pain crisis. This is pain that begins suddenly and can last hours and even days. Children with SCD often require a variety of medications, including antibiotics, pain relievers, and disease-modifying drugs. She was prescribed daily doses of Folic acid, penicillin, Hydroxyurea, Hydrocodone, and Ibuprofen very early on. In hindsight, I realize how blessed I was that my child was able to have access to treatment from birth. I could not begin to imagine how difficult it must be for families in other countries who struggle with an inadequate supply of the proper medication for this disease and others like it.

LIVING IN A BUBBLE

Our first doctor's visit to Children's Healthcare of Atlanta was quite interesting. I broke down and cried when I saw the other children who were there for similar or other life-threatening conditions. It just hit me that I'd lived in a bubble up until that point. We've been living in a bubble all our lives! You see, we wake up and go about our daily lives and worry about completing tasks we don't think twice about. We worry about trivial things. I noticed babies, toddlers, young children, and older children, some of you could tell were probably undergoing chemotherapy and other serious treatments. I felt their pain, and I just couldn't stop crying. I wasn't even thinking of my child at that moment; I was just crying more so for those kids. I began to pray and ask God, "You know what? Just forgive me. Forgive us for whining about the simplest things."

You know, money means nothing without good health. Health is wealth. We have a lot to be thankful for. That hit home for me, and I realized that, "this is what it is." I didn't even entertain the thought of what our lives would be like had Saraya not been born with SCD. The future also never crossed my mind because all I was thinking of was being there at that hospital with my daughter at present. I looked at my baby, and I looked at all those other kids, and they were kids who had been at the hospital even long before we had arrived. I thought to myself, "This is what their lives are. Who knows if they're in even worse situations than we are?" That was my empathy, the reason for my tears.

"No matter how much money you have in this world, you can't buy health. If you can't enjoy your money, it means nothing. If you are healthy, you are richer than the millionaire who is unhealthy."

The surgery for Saraya's cleft palate went well. I was distraught because of what she had to go through, but I knew we were in good hands at Children's. When you are there in the hospital room, and you see your baby with tubes in her mouth and nose, you just feel so helpless and you understand that life is so fragile.

My older children, Yakoub and Amaka, were very cooperative. Whenever my youngest was admitted to the hospital, they wanted to be there with us as a family. I remember the first time they saw the hospital, they exclaimed, "Oh mom, this looks like a kids' hotel!"

They had fun board games and video games. They make it easier and attempt to lessen the mental pain because they know what parents have to go through. I've noticed that most huge childrens' hospitals are made in such a way as to make you comfortable while you are there for your child or loved one. I'm just so appreciative. My kids were always so excited to be there with Saraya, and it didn't matter that we were all in that little room together; they loved it.

I remember on one of our stays at the hospital during the holidays, I noticed a young boy zipping down the hallway rolling on his IV stand in his hospital gown. He had to be about 8 years old. I thought to myself, " kids just want to be well and feel no pain." It is that simple; whether they have a blood disorder, cancer, leukemia, or another illness, that's all they want for Christmas. If you can take their pain away, they're fine with that. Just a chance to feel normal. That was such an eye-opening moment.

As parents, our focus is on the process of juggling work, life, and all that we have to do on a day-to-day basis. I also noticed that some kids were there for longer periods, which could be a strain on the family, so we considered ourselves quite lucky. Our stays could range from a few days to a couple of weeks in comparison to some who had been there for months. We had a lot to be grateful for.

BREAKING THE NEWS TO FAMILY

In African culture, when you have a child, everyone's waiting to hear that everything is okay. Suddenly you come and you say, "oh well, we have a baby, but the baby has…"

They start wanting to know, "well, how come?"

I remember when I first told my parents after she was born. I reluctantly told my mom she had sickle cell, and she didn't show much reaction, just a pause. On the other hand, the first thing my dad said was, "where did that come from?"

I said, "Daddy, that means I have the trait."

He said, "I don't know about that. No one in our family has that."

I was surprised at his response but decided not to let that bother me. I didn't want to end up arguing with him about it. Quite honestly, I saw it as ignorance on his part because he probably didn't know much about the disease. I only wanted them to know and suggested that they get tested to see if they have the trait. Unfortunately, my family can be stubborn, and it fell on deaf ears.

Years later, while discussing my results further with my mother, she disclosed to me that one of my cousins on her side of the family had passed away from complications of SCD. I concluded that she must have the trait.

Over the years, even though my family knew I was in and out of the hospital with my daughter, I'm not certain that they understood the magnitude or seriousness of her condition. I mean, how could they understand?

Before writing this book I had read of how there's a stigma in certain tribes in Africa amongst families and particularly women who have kids that have sickle cell. It all began to make sense to me. I wondered if that explained my father's reaction to my unexpected news. I never asked him. It's sad because from what I had read, it causes financial strain and the fathers opt to get traditional medicine for their children, not because it works, but because it's much cheaper. Some of the fathers even leave, because they can't handle the stress. Women most especially have to deal with the illness. They get the brunt of the situation because they, as caregivers, mostly work full-time and also have the responsibility of taking their kids to the hospital when they're in a crisis.

Not only that, I can only imagine it causes a strain in marriages and relationships amongst siblings as well. This is because if you have to focus more on one kid, the other siblings will sometimes feel neglected, so it takes a toll on the whole family.

I was fortunate to have children who didn't ever get jealous of or feel neglected by my attention to Saraya. Her older sister, Amaka, would say that she wished she could take her place so she could take away her pain. She hates to see her in so much pain. Yacoub was also sympathetic to her condition; he's understanding even moreso, because he's also a carrier.

I think that as a society, we need to do a lot more with helping people to understand what the illness is, what it entails, and why it is the way it is. SCD is a blood disorder, and currently, the only cure is a bone marrow or stem cell transplant. Even with that, there still may be some complications, but at least people can live longer lives as a result of it. SCD awareness is not something that should be taboo. Children with SCD may face social stigma and discrimination due to their disease. Caregivers need to advocate for their child's rights and ensure that they receive fair treatment and access to education, employment, and healthcare.

One of the many things I've discovered from my experience with SCD is that before now, I felt I was somewhat living a sheltered life. I had never experienced anything like this. Now I have become more informed, and I have counseled my kids on the importance of genetic counseling. My daughter, Amaka, got tested with her husband prior to having my grandson. I strongly advise everyone to make sure they get tested before getting married and having children to see if they have the trait.

People on the outside looking in will more than likely not understand the full scope of what you're going through. These people are also "living in a bubble," because they're often unaware of the challenges families endure when caring for a loved one and the strain it may have on family dynamics. Sometimes, you feel depleted, concerned, stressed out, and frustrated, but you continue. Being a caregiver often means giving 24 hours of one's time to care for another. It requires the dedication of time and energy. Not many people understand how strenuous it can be. Most times one has to keep a happy face and pretend all is well so that it does not affect the rest of the family.

REFLECTIONS:

Have you ever experienced this, where you've pretended you were okay at a time you weren't okay? In what ways can you relinquish control and practice asking for help once a week?

____

____

____

____

____

____

____

____

BLOOD IS LIFE

CHAPTER 3

During my prenatal visits when I was pregnant with Saraya, they gave us the usual paperwork along with a brochure on preserving the umbilical cord. It was linked to something about stem cells. I found it interesting, but at the time, I didn't think it was necessary, especially when they said it would cost about $200 for the procedure.

Back then, I didn't think much of it because I didn't have a full understanding of its benefits. The whole premise was that they would preserve the umbilical cord to be used in the future should I need it for any medical reasons. It had never crossed my mind that I would ever need it.

> ## TIP
>
> **Always do your due diligence and research any information that's presented to you, especially when it comes to your health and the health of your loved ones.**

After Saraya's birth and her diagnosis with sickle cell, we were talking to the doctor, and she explained the implications of living with SCD and what our lives would be like down the road; we were told that she would experience intense pain amongst other things. We were presented with options in which we could either do a bone marrow transplant, stem cell therapy treatment, or participate in future research opportunities.

They also mentioned that some people use the umbilical cord- cord blood banking. That was an aha moment because it made me think back to the reasoning behind the preservation of the umbilical cord. Now, in hindsight, if I had known how valuable it could have been for my daughter, I would have kept the umbilical cord. Do you see? I now know the importance and the science behind what they were offering.

Then I remember commenting at the time to the doctor. I said, "you know what? They should make cord blood banking mandatory."

Can you imagine if I had kept the umbilical cord?! Of course, it would be a different story. As I later on discovered from researching over the internet, the blood left in the umbilical cord after your baby is born is rich in stem cells. These cells help the growth and repair of body tissue. In the body, they can turn into many different cell types including blood cells, bones, cartilage, and other tissue. I would have used it on my baby! I believe that women should consider preserving their umbilical cords. An umbilical cord blood transplant, coupled with a reduced intensity conditioning (RIC) regimen, can safely and effectively treat children with genetic disorders that include sickle cell disease (SCD) and thalassemia. You just never know what the future holds, and it's best to be cautious.

Sickle cell disease is an inherited blood disorder that causes red blood cells to shrink and break down, becoming sickled or shriveled, as I like to call it. The cells die early leaving a shortage of healthy red blood cells (known as sickle cell anemia) and can block blood flow thereby causing pain (crises). It affects people of African descent, Hispanic, South Asian, southern European, and middle eastern ancestry.

Symptoms of the disease are decreased immunity to infections, extreme pain, and fatigue. There are several types of sickle cell, the most common are sickle cell anemia (SS), sickle hemoglobin - C (SC), sickle beta-plus thalassemia, and sickle beta-zero thalassemia.

Sickle cell is a genetic disorder. To get a better understanding of it, imagine a healthy red blood cell being around. Look at that as your normal blood platelet that carries oxygen inside of it. In comparison, a sickled blood cell looks shriveled. It's not as healthy as the normal platelet because it doesn't carry oxygen.

With SCD, your body is constantly making blood cells, but they are unhealthy and dying. The sickling blood platelets gather in certain parts of the body, like your joints, and they don't carry enough oxygen to your organs. So now, what happens? Well, blood is life. Blood flows to all the organs in your body, and enables your organs to function. If blood is unable to reach the necessary organs, you could end up losing these organs. Sickle cell disease can damage organs such as the spleen, liver, kidneys, and lungs. Some patients lose their spleen and gallbladder, and it could cause nerve damage, blindness, brain damage, etc. Some other complications of SCD may include organ damage, stroke, pulmonary hypertension, blindness, leg ulcers, gallstones, and splenic sequestration. Each year, Saraya has a brain scan to make sure there's no nerve damage.

SCD can cause pain in the bones, joints, and abdomen. The pain episodes, also known as sickle cell crises, can be triggered by stress, infection, dehydration, and other factors. When the sickled cells travel through the small blood vessels, they can get stuck and clog the blood flow. This is what causes the pain. Imagine continuous intense sharp throbbing pain. Saraya describes it as blood not flowing through her joints. Signs of a crisis can include swelling of the joints, frequent infections, vision problems, and extreme pain. This can last from hours to days to weeks. Anything can trigger a sickle cell crisis, such as a change in temperature, strenuous exercise, dehydration, stress, high altitudes, smoking, and alcohol consumption. It can be stress-related, whether emotional, mental, or physical.

We could be happy-go-lucky one minute and the next thing we know, she is in pain, and she has to be taken to the ER. The pain could be anywhere, from her neck to her chest, her joints, or her legs. It would be extreme to the point where sometimes she couldn't walk. She would constantly scream in pain. The drill is to give her pain medication - Ibuprofen and Hydrocodone, every 4 to 6 hours. If she is still in pain, I call the doctor on-call and let them know I am bringing her in.

Sitting in that waiting room, I would ponder to myself. I knew God had prepared me for such a time as this, and the same would ring true even on those long nights when I had to drive to the emergency room, almost falling asleep at the wheel. It would usually be at odd times of the day, mostly at midnight. I'd be driving and praying for Jesus to take the wheel, so that we get there safely with no mishaps.

In the ER, if there's still no breakthrough with her pain crises and her red blood cell counts are low, then she may need to get a blood transfusion.

There's a huge transformation when she receives a transfusion. It's like she becomes alive. This lends truth to the saying that "blood is life."

The first time Saraya got a blood transfusion, she was two years old. I was very cautious as a parent because of her condition. The main reason for the transfusion was that her hemoglobin levels were low. I remember praying on it and saying, "you know what? This is what life is like."

I said, "please God, just let this flow through her and let it rejuvenate her." Whenever she takes the transfusion, she's like a new person, so full of life and energy! I felt relieved when I saw the instant change in her health. In the subsequent transfusions she's had over the years, I'd always tell her, "you know, you're like a vampire because then you become alive!" She finds that so funny.

Luckily, she hasn't had very many transfusions since she was two years old. Another thing I noticed is that no two individuals are alike when it comes to how the body handles the disease. You may have two individuals with the same diagnosis, but the way their body handles it is completely different.

I can tell when she's about to have a crisis; her eyes become slightly yellow and she's lethargic and tired. Once she gets a blood transfusion, her eyes are all clear. She's just vibrant! That's why I always say "blood is life."

As a caregiver, I have to keep up with all her medications and doctor visits, which can be over-whelmingly strenuous and challenging considering that I juggled that with my demanding full-time job. As Saraya grew older, I also had to make sure that she took her medication. There were times when she would hide her medication. I remember seeing a bunch of pills underneath my bed at one point. I got angry, because I was frustrated with the fact that I thought I was doing my best to keep her healthy and believed that she was cooperating with me.

Though my initial reaction was to scold her, I thought twice and tried to put myself in her shoes to understand what she was going through. She had been on medication for so long that she was getting frustrated. She was always sick and felt like the med-ication wasn't helping her, so she decided she didn't want to take it anymore. On top of that, she was stressed and worried that she constantly had to miss school. It was such a difficult time for her. She told me she just didn't care anymore. I decided to have her speak with a therapist whenever we went in to see her doctor.

Caregiving requires an enormous amount of compassion for the individual, especially in circumstances where you have to take care of the person for an indefinite period of time. It does take a toll on the caregiver as one begins to feel a sense of hopelessness and one wonders if one is capable of sustaining the lifestyle. Talk about compassion fatigue!

Compassion fatigue has been described as the convergence of secondary traumatic stress (STS) and cumulative burnout (BO), a state of physical and mental exhaustion caused by a depleted ability to cope with one's everyday environment.

It is so important to communicate with the loved one you are caring for (their feelings and experiences, as well as yours). I cannot stress this enough. Most times, we feel we know everything that is going on with our loved ones. You will be amazed at how much of a disconnect there is because you never took the time to talk or have them express themselves. As caregivers, we can get so caught up in trying to 'fix' things and fail to listen to what's going on with our loved ones on a deeper level.

Because SCD is often accompanied by severe, unpredictable pain crises, it can be difficult to manage. Caregivers need to work closely with healthcare providers to develop a pain management plan that can help relieve the child's discomfort. Children with SCD often require a variety of medications, including antibiotics, pain relievers, and disease-modifying drugs. Caregivers need to ensure that their child takes their medications as prescribed and manage any side effects.

Saraya takes Hydroxyurea, which helps with managing the pain crises and she's able to take it with no adverse side effects. Folic acid helps with increasing iron in her blood, aids in transporting oxygen throughout her body, and is important for red blood cell formation and healthy cell growth and function. Penicillin helps to protect her immune system. It keeps her from contracting any infection. Hydrocodone-acetaminophen and Ibuprofen help to relieve pain and fevers in most cases. She also takes Albuterol, as needed, it is a breathing treatment that helps with Acute chest syndrome. Acute chest syndrome is a complication of sickle cell disease that could be life-threatening; it occurs when sickled cells clump together in the lungs.

When Saraya was a toddler, I could tell she was having a pain crisis when she would moan through her sleep and develop high fevers. Having high fevers means constant visits to the ER at unexpected times to figure out what triggered the change. Even to this day, a high fever means everything stops for me, and she becomes my main focus.

The unpredictability of the pain crises is what gets to me. Just when I think I can take a breather and sit back to relax and take on personal projects, that brief moment is short-lived by her screams of pain. My plan of action is to administer her pain meds. If that doesn't work and it only gets worse with her screaming, then I know we're in for a long night. If she has a fever, I call the hospital. The doctor on-call asks me to bring her in. I look at the clock. It's 11 p.m. or 12 midnight, and I'm half asleep. I begrudgingly get up and pack an overnight bag because I know that once we get admitted, I don't like leaving her alone. That, my friends, is just a snippet of what we have to deal with when handling pain crises.

I don't know how I managed, but there were countless times that I had to do this, even while working a full-time job. There were times when I'd almost hit the guardrail on the highway.

I cannot tell you how I physically survived, but I'm telling you that when God has a purpose for you, he preserves and keeps you from harm. He provides that shield and covering over you. And nothing, I mean nothing can get in the way. Anything could have happened, you know? Lucky for me, my teenage kids were in high school and understood the severity of their sister's condition so they were able to at least take care of themselves. They did the right thing, so I didn't have to worry much about my home being in a mess; they helped and I'm so grateful for their understanding.

REFLECTIONS:

How have you been able to push through? What are some things you may have taken for granted that you appreciate more than ever since you've become a caregiver?

____

____

____

____

____

____

____

____

PATIENTS NEED OUTLETS TO FEEL ALIVE

CHAPTER 4

When Saraya was eight years old I gave her a necklace as a coping mechanism because she was having separation anxiety. She would cry every time before leaving home for school. When I would ask her what was wrong, she would say, "Well, I don't want to leave you."

I would respond by telling her, "well, this is just school."

I assured her that when she got back, I'd still be here, but that didn't ever seem to help. She would always cry. That was when a thought occurred to me to give her something of mine which she could hold on to kind of like how Kevin Costner would give his clients in The Bodyguard movie (although there was no tracking device attached to it). She loved the idea.

The necklace I gifted her had a horse on it. My name, Philippa, means "lover of horses." I told her to wear it and touch it when thinking of me or when she felt alone and to look at that horse and know that I am with her.

MAKING FRIENDS

When she was in the first grade, she made friends with twin sisters and they played a pivotal part in her life. She had problems making friends because she missed school frequently. The twins lived close by which made it easy for them to connect, and they became the best of friends. Usually, Saraya wouldn't entertain sleepovers, but she was comfortable hanging with the twins.

She met her twin friends in elementary school, and they'd been friends for a couple of years leading up to when they started middle school. They were quite close. She would go trick-or-treating with them and just hang out, and I was thrilled she had friends she had connected with in that way.

Having a social life can be difficult for the patients as well as caregivers. Most kids grapple with what to tell their friends or how to explain what they're going through. The other kids may not understand, and that leaves the kid with the burden of having to keep explaining themselves if they fail to meet obligations. There were times when Saraya would go for a sleepover or even just a visit, and then I'd get a phone call saying that she was having a crisis or that she was in pain. I would have to drop everything to go get her. It always seemed to be that way. There was never a moment where she would stay through an event. At times I wondered if it was a combination of separation anxiety and her crises. Interestingly, I believe that separation anxiety causes her stress, which also leads to pain crises.

If I'm honest, when she visited with friends, I couldn't relax because I knew at any moment I would get a phone call to come to get her. I had to be "on call" just in case. I would have loved to be able to take some time for myself but somehow I could never seem to relax because I always anticipated she would need me. This is a constant for the caregiver; we feel that infinite weight of responsibility for our loved ones. So can you imagine when they become adults? Are we willing or ready to let go? That's another stage in this caregiver journey because I think as caregivers, we need to trust that our loved ones can live their lives independently. It's easier said than done, but that's a struggle we face.

THE LETTER

When she was in first grade, I attended Saraya's end-of-the-year class presentation, where parents are invited to see what their children have worked on throughout the school year. That was the year her dad moved back to Nigeria. I remember Saraya presented a letter she wrote that hit me hard. She was letting me know that she was afraid of losing me since her dad had left. She didn't want me to leave. The letter touched me. I remember a mother was sitting beside me, unknowingly expressing her pity for my daughter as she said, "oh how sad". I thought to myself, "oh God, here we go". In that very short moment, I felt embarrassed as a mother. The letter addressed her insecurities, her frustrations, and especially her fears.

She is very reserved and she doesn't talk much, so I was quite surprised and impressed with her writing. It was a good thing to hear her thoughts at that age and understand what she was feeling. And, I guess that would be the beginning of many more of what I affectionately like to call her... "rants." She wasn't expressing herself in a bad way, but from within, what she was truly feeling. She has evolved as time has passed, expressing her emotions through her music and songwriting. It's been beautiful to be able to witness her write her truth.

Over the years, she's continued to express her feelings and even her siblings have noticed her tenacity. They are amazed at her progress and creativity. Her songs depict the pain she constantly has to deal with. Her sister Amaka once asked me, "Are you paying attention to the lyrics?"

To which I responded, "Yeah, I know. She's allowed to express herself. What's wrong with self-expression?"

She further added, "Oh, don't you think she should speak to a therapist?"

I understand her siblings are concerned about her emotional and mental wellbeing, but I tell them that we all need an outlet to express our emotions. She uses her music to let the outside world know what she's experiencing on the inside.

Being a single parent. I've always taught my kids to be open with me. My kids find it easy to talk to me whenever they have any problems. When their dad left, I assured them that they were my priority. Most times when I'm tired and frustrated, they can see it. Even still, I try to be available when they need me. I've always been big on communication. It is extremely important to consider the feelings of others because it is easy to get caught up in our frustration and forget that at the end of the day, it's nothing personal. People express themselves based on their experiences and the only way they know how.

It can get frustrating for the caregiver when they're constantly reminded of the mental or emotional state of their loved one. It almost feels as if we are incompetent or not doing enough for those in our care… Because, how could we?

As a caregiver, having time for yourself is a luxury. At the back of your mind, you are overwhelmed with feeling guilty that you're ignoring your patient. I have never entertained the thought of regret like, "Oh, I wish I wouldn't have put her in this situation." As a parent, we should be cautious of the words we use to express guilt because children may misconstrue that to mean, "Oh, so I wasn't meant to be?" Things like that can negatively tamper with their psyche. There's no such thing as a mistake. There are no coincidences.

The letter Saraya wrote in class gave me an insight into her resilience and how smart and intelligent she really is. It gave me a glimpse into her character; I learned that my shy daughter is very outspoken. She may be quiet, but she's strong-willed.

I believe everything happens for a reason, just like when she was born. I've never questioned the fact that she has sickle cell. The responsibility falls on us to accept and make the best of the lives we have. I've never questioned God about our circumstances.

As much as things would probably have seemed less stressful without our family experiencing this illness upfront and personally, I believe it's not always about me. This is a lesson within itself. It involves growing as an individual. It's an experience. It's how you look at that experience. There's a lesson to be learned in all of this, whether it is doing one's due diligence to gain compassion in its purest form, or working on self-development. Each day this experience is making me stronger, pulling from me something I never knew I had before now, or how much I was capable of handling. It's not just my daughter's burden, but my lesson too. I'm learning each day.

As I mentioned earlier, being that she was always absent from school, I believe making new friends was difficult for Saraya. She's a very private person. This illness keeps her even more secluded. It's not like she didn't talk to her classmates or other people, but for the most part, she keeps to herself. Through it all, her teachers had only good things to say about her.

Imagine being in school and feeling so tired you are unable to do simple things like running or playing with your friends. It wasn't that she was incapable of being active; she was a very fast runner. That's the funny thing. In her mind and her body, she knew what she was capable of doing but because of her ailment, she was restricted. That can be frustrating! Even when she would want to sign up for certain activities, she was unable to follow through with and complete them due to her crises. At the time, I felt it would not be wise to even sign her up for activities knowing she couldn't follow through. She always had to be careful not to overexert herself because she also has Acute chest syndrome. It's one of the side effects of sickle cell that affects the lungs to the point where she finds it difficult to breathe.

HER DETERMINATION TO WIN

Even so, I noticed Saraya was determined to win something at school. Because she noticed her older siblings had received academic awards at school over the years, she was bent on winning something. I told her regardless, to me, she was my hero. Being able to get good grades in school despite her illness was in itself an amazing feat.

She still took part in the year-end school races and finally won a medal for a 50-yard dash in 4th grade. Before the race, I told her, "we know you can run. You are a fighter. I know what you're capable of doing, so you don't have to prove anything to any-one. Only do this for yourself."

As caregivers, we should encourage our loved ones to try to live 'normal' lives and not hold them back from their dreams or aspirations.

GIVING HER A COMMUNITY OF HER OWN

I'd been thinking of ways to keep Saraya connected with her peers, and I'd been hearing of this sickle cell camp called Camp New Hope, but at that time, I think I was waiting for her to get a bit older. When the right time came, I suggested it to her. I said, "you know what? I think you need to see other kids," thinking it'd be a good idea for her to meet someone else who had the same condition as her, "I think it's about time you went camping because that's a way for you to get out of the house."

I needed her to see that she wasn't alone and for her to improve her social skills. I felt this was the perfect chance for her to mix with other kids that shared the same medical condition.

I applaud the camp administration and staff because it really is good for the kids. In addition to being good for the kids, it's also beneficial for the parents, because as a caregiver, you then have time to yourself. I'll be honest though. The very first time she went, I was somewhat concerned. The camp lasted for a week, and they advised the parents to write letters to their children each day. When I sent her off, I put my letters in a bag and handed them over to the administrators. They were labeled for each day of the week.

In each letter, I would tell her how proud I was of her, but I never mentioned that I missed her, because I didn't want her to get worried. Remember, she was already battling separation anxiety, so I didn't want to add any other factor that might feed her anxiety. So I would write, "you know what? Today was a good day. How was your day today? I'm super proud of you."

I would encourage her and hype her up in every letter. Another thing was that I never called. Once she was gone, that was it. That was my way of cutting the umbilical cord. That's not to say that I didn't miss her; the days went by fast. And on the last day when I picked her up, I made sure I arrived early to get her. She was excited to see me, and I could tell that she had evolved mentally in such a short time. I could see that she made friends; everyone was saying, " Hey Saraya! Bye Saraya! I'll see you!"

We discussed the trip beforehand. I said, "okay, you're going off to camp. There are no phone calls. Even if you are allowed to call, I'm not going to call you, because it's your time for yourself. This is my time to myself, and I know you'll be back.

I didn't mention that I was going to miss her. I didn't want her to start thinking of that. After the fact, when she came back home, she told me she missed me. I said, "yeah, I know. Same thing here, but I wasn't going to tell you, 'I miss you.'"

I didn't tell her verbally because I knew it would have stuck in her mind the whole trip. I knew for a fact she was having fun, and that helped. I set the parameters before she left and explained how things would be. I pulled back and told her, I'm not calling you. They said 'no phones,' so no cell phones."

When she came back, she said, "like you said, 'no phones,' but there were kids there with their phones."

I said, "well, that's them. You didn't have to do it. It didn't kill you. You're back. It was just 7 days. It worked out."

That was such a positive thing. Sometimes we underestimate our loved ones, thinking, "oh, they wouldn't manage." Trust me, the first two days in a new camp environment, kids are trying to find themselves. That's what we all do when we're faced with a new challenge, right? They were able to immerse themselves in all the activities. Of course, the camp organizers give them so much to do, along with teaching them how to cope with their pain. I feel like that was a good thing. I also told her that she could someday be a counselor helping other kids. I let her know that almost every one of them had sickle cell so she wasn't the only one.

My hope when I signed her up for the summer camp was that she could see that she was not alone and that other kids and individuals were battling the same condition.

MY ANXIETY

I often experience feelings of anxiety, guilt, and helplessness. This can happen when going through life changes such as when my older kids were going off to college. I worried about how they would manage college life. I had terrible thoughts of receiving dreaded phone calls that they were in danger. The mind is a very powerful tool. I prayed and asked God to protect them because they were out of my hands. I let God take control. He gave me a certain peace about the whole situation.

This is a coping mechanism I use to manage stress and anxiety. When I anticipate difficult changes, I begin to prepare myself mentally. I also try to stay positive and motivated. Lately, I have included positive self-talk. I remind myself not to sweat the small stuff. I try not to focus or dwell on trivial matters because, at the end of the day, it is nothing personal. I also advise my children to find ways to manage their emotions.

THE POWER OF MUSIC

During the COVID-19 pandemic, Saraya developed an interest in playing the electric guitar after watching her brother play. Of course when she had pain crises, I encouraged her to bring her guitar with her to the hospital. I knew it would help to make her happy.

Saraya's music has become an outlet for her to express whatever she's going through and her pain. That is her happy place. On one of our hospital stays, she was able to take her instrument. On another occasion, she would take her drawing pad. Anything to help take her mind off the pain.

When I discovered her love for music, I decided to support her. I bought her some instruments, two electric guitars, an amplifier, and an electric drum set. We set up a mini studio. She records her music and has released songs online as well. Of course, she lets me listen to her beats and I have my favorites. Some of the best ones she's written were when she was at the hospital. I was amazed!

Here's the lyrics to one of her songs below.

Untitled
You can't be understood. I tell, still no good.

I hate the way you make me drowsy, all for control
The way one single task could trigger, understood
If only you could know, I have some goals.
You have me chained, always maybe forever.
You can be so difficult for no reason.
The days I missed, you cause the pressure.
I hate how you ruin the best seasons.

You can be as bitter as the winter
You give no rest nor do the others have it best.
But I know your ways, you're quite the hinter.
One wrong move, I'm put to test; now I'm stressed.

(TRICKY)
Verse:
If only you know that I too have goals
Enough is enough
You have me,
Chained in vain
Restricted in pain
Enough is enough
You have me in locked up

Chorus:
And you can be as bitter as the winter
Yeah, you give me no rest nor do the others have
it best but…
I know your ways you're quite the hinter

One wrong move I'm put to the test, now I'm
stressed
One move, your triggered
And I should've figured
No cure it's understood

Verse:
If only I knew that I wasn't few
Enough is enough
The truth is in,
View, it true
This life ain't so blue
I run through the dew I feel so brand new

Bridge:
I'm drowsy for control
Truth be told
And it's all that you know
When your own
And just hold me close
That's all I need the most
The new day is over the horizon
I see it from these clean white walls
That cot

Interestingly, I've stumbled on a couple of writings by
kids suffering from sickle cell and how they refer to

the pain crises as "the beast." This couldn't be far from the truth.

Her lyrics sum it all up as confronting, battling, and overcoming this beast - pain crises. She portrays some really deep emotions. I get it though. And to me, it's okay for her to express herself however she deems fit. When her sister listened to her song, she said to me, "have you listened to Saraya's song?"

I said, "yes, I have. I don't find anything wrong with it. Hey, artists paint. They paint their pain and their agony. What's wrong with that? That's a way to let it out. We express ourselves in different ways. I think it's interesting because someone out there can relate to what she's going through."

I told Saraya when she started this journey with music that at some point she would need to decide what she wanted to do with her talent. I told her that no one should change the narrative of what she is writing and to be true to herself. "You don't need to answer to anyone; just express yourself. It's okay. Trust me. There is an audience out there that will appreciate what you have to say. Now, if you want to be commercial, then you do what everyone else is doing. And you'll go commercial. You stay true to who you are."

There are times when I feel as though I give so much of myself making sure my loved ones are okay. I have to remember to take care of my emotional well-being. I keep a small circle of friends and I try to check in with family. Once in a while, I make time to meet up for lunch or a girls' outing. I also have a significant other who is there for me when I need to talk.

Interestingly enough my oldest daughter, Amaka, thinks that my personality has rubbed off on Saraya in that I can be a bit of a recluse. When Saraya was younger, I stayed home quite a bit. But now I'm mentally preparing myself because I know that there will be some changes soon. That big thing is the anticipation of her leaving home. She's getting older, and we are getting to the point where she's going to be on her own.

I feel as if I've lived my life in survival mode for so many years. That's just the way it is, always on edge. I found that even when I want to take a breather, even something as simple as relaxing in my bed and reading a book, something always comes up. When that happens multiple times, in the end, I just resign myself to the fact, "what else is going to happen?". That's just how I get by. It's gotten a bit better, but I find that my mindset is still in survival mode. It's not just concerning Saraya but also my older ones. If they need help and they reach out to me, I have to do all that I can to be available for them. On the other hand, I remind myself that there'll come a time when I feel like I'm no longer needed. That's when one will have to figure out what is one's purpose and how to get on with life. That's what a lot of single parents go through. If your whole life has been built around your children and suddenly they are grown and leave home, you then have to figure out what you're going to do with yourself.

Some years ago I started creating little moments. We would go to the beach for the weekend. Saraya loves the water and surfing. I try to do at least one trip a year to get out of the city.

During the pandemic, we thought of taking a trip to Seattle. Saraya had mentioned that she would love to move to Seattle and go to school there. I asked her "why Seattle of all places?"

She said she loves the weather. I told her that it rains a lot there. She said she loves the rain. Needless to say, Seattle remains on our bucket list. The only stipulation was that she wanted us to go together as a family, not just with only me because I can tend to be boring.

REFLECTIONS:

What are some lessons you're learning as you go through this experience? What good can you pull from this? How has this impacted your life in positive ways? What's your silver lining?

____

____

____

____

____

____

____

____

____

DISRUPTION CALLS FOR A REALITY CHECK

CHAPTER 5

So this was one of those moments, one of those extended stays at the hospital, we had gone because she had this terrible crisis. We were staying there longer than usual. During that time, the hospital had arranged for us caregivers and parents to meet and talk about what we were going through. That was the first and only time I'd ever attended one of those meet-and-greets. It helped me to see the other parents and what they were talking about. I was in awe hearing the different experiences each had and didn't know things like this happened. Some parents spoke of not having a social life, and some shared difficulties when traveling by air because high altitudes are not good for sicklers (that was a new term to me). Even though I knew other families had kids with sickle cell, I was just in my head about our situation, not understanding the full scope of what others were going through.

I remember meeting this particular lady. She told me about her daughter, and I asked her if she would be open to having her daughter speak to my daughter before they checked out of the hospital. We had been there for about a day, and our daughters were just about the same age. I went back to the hospital room and I told my daughter, "Hey, guess what? I have someone I'd like you to meet."

Usually, when we're on admission, we rarely mingle with the other patients so she was hesitant. She usually doesn't care to have anyone else there except for close family.

She said, "no, I don't want to."

I wasn't thinking about the pain she was in. Even though she was on her pain medication, she was still in pain. When they're having pain crises they can come off as being obnoxious or angry at times, but they have all the reasons to. They're going through something other people cannot understand, so she just didn't want to talk to or see anyone. Either way, I managed to convince her, I told her, "well, I think you need to speak with this girl. She's just about your age."

That turned out to be a revealing moment for us both. For the first time, I heard how Saraya felt about her sickness. She said she questioned why it had to be her. She also thought she was the only one in the world going through this ordeal.

When we're in the hospital, I get frustrated especially when Saraya and I have those arguments over trivial things where we go back and forth after being cooped up in the hospital for so long. She breaks down crying, and I'm like, "you know what? That's kind of uncalled for on my part. It's not all about me." At that moment, I have to put myself in her situation and be considerate. We are over-whelmed with all these emotions and it'd be nice to have an outlet to vent about it all. As much as we're allowed to vent, we may never really understand what our loved ones go through.

As caregivers, we are selfless with our time be-cause we know that our loved ones look to us for care and comfort. Her aunt has offered to stay with her on numerous occasions. Honestly, I would re-fuse because I didn't want it to be the last time that I saw my daughter. I don't want to feel like I was away from her and missed a moment with her. There have been times when her aunt would plead with me to leave, but I just found it much too difficult to leave her side.

I'd just tell her, "that won't be necessary. I'd ra-ther be here."

As I mentioned earlier staying cooped up for days in the hospital room can be tedious and frus-trating for us both because of the amount of mor-phine in her system, she starts to itch or she gets angry and frustrated. When that happens, we start arguing. During these moments I have to put on my big girl pants and get out of my head to see things her way. It's nothing personal; I try not to make it about me.

Well, the smart thing for me to do would be to leave the room and take some time off. My sister-in-law would offer to watch her while I take a breather. I'm usually reluctant to do so. The guilt trip kicks in and I'm thinking, "What if I leave and find out something happened and I wasn't there?" That's why I find it difficult to leave. To just walk out that door and something unexpected happens without me having the chance to say goodbye. I get emotional thinking about it.

Yes, I do get frustrated. Yes, I'm allowed to get frustrated. It's okay. I'm human. And I get over it. These are valid feelings. These are things we have to go through as caregivers.

On one occasion, I got so frustrated because I felt Saraya wasn't following instructions regarding her medication. When she's on morphine, sometimes they give her this pump with a button she has to press to administer her small dose. When she feels pain, she's supposed to press the button. Well with the way the medication works on the body, she's always falling asleep, so she may not remember to push it. Sometimes she'd be awake, but she would just choose not to press it. And in my mind, I'm screaming, "well, you are the one in pain. Do something!"

I'm not trying to be inconsiderate, but maybe it's mental. Our argument would go something like this...

Me: You need to press your pump.

Saraya: Mom, I'm trying (rolling her eyes).

Me: You are supposed to push the button when it turns green. I don't think you're trying hard enough.

Saraya: (remains silent)

Me: Okay, you know what? I need to take some time away.

Saraya: No, please don't go.

Her older sister once said, "you guys are just like sisters bickering because you stay with each other 24/7."

I said, "yeah, but that's my life. There is no complaining."

Life is short, so enjoy what you can. And that's the reason why when I go to the hospital if she's in a crisis and we pack her bags, that's it. I'm locked in.

JUGGLING CORPORATE AMERICA AND HEALTH

For a while when she'd experience these episodes, I would take time off from work. Then there came a time when I had to let my supervisors at work know because my work was beginning to suffer. They knew that she has sickle cell and that I was struggling with it affecting my work, and they were somewhat supportive. The only time I would take off work would be if she had a crisis. Once I get out of the hospital, it's really hard trying to get back into my work routine. It kind of chipped away at me.

It's difficult to avoid falling into some kind of depression. For the longest, I knew I was battling it; I just didn't want to express it or say it because I didn't want it to be held against me. That's another thing we struggle with as caregivers. I believe that most caregivers, especially women, constantly worry about whether the employer will question their ability to do the job they are hired to do. I knew I was competent, but I was worried that if I mentioned this, it would be used against me. Even though I'd been with that company for about 7 years, I just didn't want to be seen as someone that wasn't able to do my job. I knew the magnitude of what I was going through, and I just needed some time to deal with my health issues. In hindsight, I don't know if that's a good or a bad thing, because we do have resources. I could have talked to a therapist. I could have joined a support group for caregivers.

Having that emotional support is so vital.

Caregivers also need to educate their child's school about the disease to ensure that the child receives appropriate care and support. At the beginning of each school year, I had a meeting with the principal and her teachers to brief them about her condition and explain to them that there would be school absences. I also made sure the school knew to call me if Saraya was having a crisis so that I could pick her up. There were quite several times when that happened and I would have to leave work. I had already spoken to Saraya and assured her that if she ever felt anything, it was okay to go to the nurse's office and have them call me. So everyone was aware. It was important for me to do my due diligence.

My job allowed me to work remotely. I have a reserved personality. With Saraya being born with her condition, I just didn't want to be around people much. I didn't see the joy in being around others at that time. I would avoid social functions at all costs.

Utilizing my resources would have been a move in a great direction though, a start to prioritize myself and my well-being. Sadly, oftentimes the focus is solely on getting the job done no matter what. That's the hand we're dealt as women, especially as single moms. We worry about whether or not we're doing a good job at juggling it all. So for the longest, I just kept going. That's what I knew to do. I put a smile on my face and kept it moving. I hid behind that facade and tried my best to do what I had to do.

It was time for employee performance check-in at work, and I sat down with my supervisor to discuss my work and my goals. She made a comment that shook me.

I wasn't surprised at her level of comfort with telling me because we'd had previous conversations about life, and we were very cordial; it was just what she said that stopped me in my tracks. She said, "I do applaud you because of your situation and you do so much here at work. Are you okay? I just wanted to check up on you."

She knew about Saraya's case, and she's always expressed concern about it. She's even let me know that if I ever needed help to let her know. I believe she had the best of intentions.

She continued, "I worry so much about you because I'm telling you, I wouldn't be surprised if one day I heard that you jumped off a bridge because you have so much to handle."

I said, "whoa, whoa, whoa. Is that how you see me?"

She said, "I just worry for you because you don't talk much. You don't ask for help or anything."

I had to explain to her that it was because I'm in survival mode. Sometimes you just don't think about stuff; you just up and do it. There are no ifs and buts about it. You don't get a break. When she said that, I was surprised. I was thinking, "whoa, is this how people look at me?"

It just reaffirmed that I was seeing myself as less than what people were seeing me as. Sometimes, as caregivers, we see ourselves as not doing enough, all the while others are perceiving us as superheroes. We tend to discount ourselves a lot. We don't focus on ourselves. We think less of what we do and what we go through. Meanwhile, others see more of what we do than we give ourselves credit for.

I know what I'm capable of and what my strengths are. My boss would always tell me that she was so impressed and amazed and felt I'm such a strong woman. She was proud of how I handled things, but her concern was that I never complained about my situation and I just continued to do my work. I wouldn't talk to people about it to the extent of depression and she could see that. All she knew is that I would show up to work and do my work. She wondered if I had anyone that I could speak to or anyone that was helping me. I tried to explain to her that sometimes when you're faced with something and you're in survival mode, you don't even second guess and think.

Because of that, I realized even more that I probably have it good. Some people are in worse situations. We each have our cross to bear. I am capable of handling my situation better than the next man. I may not be able to handle what others are handling, and vice versa. We must not discount what we have persevered through. Rather, we need to pat ourselves on the back and acknowledge how far we've come. It takes a certain level of resilience to go to battle for our loved ones. We stretch ourselves, and we need to take some time out consistently for self-love, self-care, and self-appreciation.

Having that conversation with my supervisor was a huge eye-opener. I mentioned it to my eldest daughter, Amaka, and she was like, "you know, you need to take care of yourself. I keep telling you."

It reinforced exactly what I was thinking. It's not like I didn't know I needed to take care of myself. It was just my mentality to keep going and keep working through it without stopping to think. As caregivers, there is a dire need for us to take time out to relax.

I recall a coworker had a daughter with a serious heart condition. She carried a pacemaker with her. The school would often call her because of her daughter's heart condition. She had a plan in place that if anything happened, they'd automatically transport her daughter to the hospital immediately and she would leave work to go to her daughter. When I saw firsthand her situation, I felt so grateful. The grass is never greener on the other side. Seeing what she was going through let me know that I wasn't alone. My goal is to make it comfortable for myself and comfortable for Saraya. I just take it one day at a time. I've resigned myself to the fact that this is a lifetime situation. I've met other parents with adult kids that have sickle cell who still have to be in their children's lives. My mentality has changed to the fact that I'll just take everything one day at a time and be there for my daughter. My focus right now is also on taking care of myself. Saraya also has expressed that she wants me to take care of myself and for me to be happy.

NOT SO HOT GIRL SUMMER

The summer of 2018, was one of those very very hot summers. My son, Yakoub, was still at home with us.

I asked him to mow the lawn and he didn't do it when I wanted him to. With me being who I am, I took it upon myself to just do it. While cutting the grass, I failed to hydrate myself. I knew I was thirsty, but I'm the kind of person that doesn't like to stop once I start working. I like to finish my work and then sit back and relax. That's what I had in mind. So I continued mowing the lawn in my backyard and noticed I was sweating profusely, but I thought that was normal because it was so hot. I decided to stop for a while and stepped into the house. Yakoub saw me drenched in sweat and asked, "What are you doing?!"

I said to him, "Well, I'm doing what I asked you to do."

He said, "Why are you doing that?"

I said, "Because when I ask you to do something, I expect it to be done! Not on your time, but when I tell you to."

If left to him, it would take forever, so I decided to do it myself.

He said, "Well, I told you I was going to do it."

We weren't necessarily arguing, but we were having a back-and-forth conversation. The next thing

I know, all I could think was that I couldn't catch my breath. I was trying my hardest to breathe. I didn't realize I was passing out. I had never had that happen to me before. In my mind, I thought I was still having a conversation with my son. Unknown to me, I was sliding down to the floor. My fists were clenched. I couldn't open up my palms. They were so tightly clenched. I felt myself having muscle spasms. In my mind, I was lucid. I thought I was awake and still alert.

I found out later from my son that I wasn't. He said, "No, you passed out ."

I said, "No, I could hear everything you were saying."

He said, "No, you passed out three times."

I came to find out that I had a heat stroke. I was clenching, and I thought I was telling my son, "Don't let my fists clench; don't let my body curl up. I need you to open my palms. Open my palms."

He wasn't hearing anything I was saying. I kept saying, "Help me. Help me. Call my mom. Call my mom in Brazil to pray for me. Call Daryl (my significant other). Call him. Don't let my hands clench up. It feels like I'm clenching up, and I can't move my joints. I need you to help me. Help me. Help me."

I was saying all of this, but my son couldn't hear me. The internal dialogue that was going on in my head was unknown to him. He yelled for Saraya, and they called 9-1-1. I was on the floor, and I couldn't move. I was in so much pain, and my joints ached. Saraya just stood there looking, worried. In my mind, I knew I was awake, but my son told me that I had passed out the whole time.

When the paramedics came, they asked Yakoub to get me a banana and some gatorade.

When I came to, Yacoub told me, "don't ever do that again. You passed out 3 times."

I told him that I heard everything he was saying. That was a wake-up call for me. It opened my mind so much, and I began to think so deeply. I thought of individuals in the hospital who are paralyzed from stroke and unable to speak. They are able to communicate with their eyes. It is possible their minds are alert. They can hear you, but the thing is that they are so locked in their bodies that they can't move. I couldn't stop thinking about those that are bedridden and who may be alive inside.

Weeks after my incident, my muscles were still sore. I was concerned with how that might have affected Saraya. So I asked her about it. She told me, "if anything had happened to you, I would stop talking. I would never speak again or talk to anyone."

I felt terrible for not taking good care of myself. I wouldn't be able to forgive myself if she never spoke again.

Since that day, Yakoub hasn't had any arguments with me. He tries his best not to frustrate me, because in his mind, he keeps replaying that scene over and over again, and he thinks if we argue that it may happen again. He said he was scared. When he sees me, he just tries to warn me about when I raise my voice, trying to remind me to calm down and take it easy.

REFLECTIONS:

Do the loved ones that you care for have an outlet to express themselves and/or their community of friends? What outlets and communities
make it easier for them to relate and feel seen?
What outlets/communities can bring joy and encouragement to their lives?

TIME TO STOP BEING THE VICTIM AND BECOME THE VICTOR

CHAPTER 6

One of the main things I learned about while attending a Sickle Cell conference during National Sickle Cell Awareness Month in September was being a part of a huge community and understanding that I am not alone. That there were others who were going through what I was going through. I noticed that there were people in even worse situations than I was, and it just made me even more grateful and careful with my thoughts. As human beings, we're quick to point fingers, and oftentimes, we think the grass is greener on the other side. I believe that there's a reason we're given every situation we find ourselves in. As I said before, there are no coincidences. Where we are is where we are meant to be right here and now. At the conferences, I've seen kids who are going through similar situations as Saraya is, but who are affected differently, and sometimes even worse ways than she is presently. It just makes me even more grateful for how she's handling it. We do have tough times, but I've been given what I can handle. Through these conferences, not only do I get to network with other families experiencing similar situations, but she also gets to see other kids with their families and learn about their trials and what difficulties they have. The conferences are also a place where we are introduced to all of the research and breakthroughs that are go-ing on.

She's in an enlightened stage right now because she's experiencing so much emotionally and becom-ing more aware of everything, from world events to societal problems. This is that teenage phase where some kids can be bratty. When I say "bratty," I know it's not intentional, but it's just her trying to process her emotions and what she's going through. This be-gan when she had just started high school. I could understand on an even deeper level because not only has she had to endure her illness but she had the extra layer of having to attend her first year of high school from home because of COVID-19. That was difficult. When we would go for doctors' visits, I would have her talk to a therapist to express herself, and they would give her tips on how to process her emotions.

TAKING ADVANTAGE OF RESEARCH OPPORTU-NITIES

Being a part of the research program we've joined has helped Saraya tremendously; her crises have lessened greatly. I'm not saying she doesn't have discomfort once in a while, but it's not as bad as it used to be. She's responding very well to treatment. What makes me proud about all of this is that it's something she chose on her own. Two years ago, when we were in the hospital, I was pushing more for the invasive treatment of bone marrow transplant. In my head, I thought, "well, this is one shot," but then again, there's a chance that it may not go well. So when the doctor gave us the options and she chose infusion, I said, "Okay, well that's a no-brainer."

The fact that it came from her meant so much to me. I didn't choose it. She chose what she thought would be best for her. I think that's a good thing, depending on your child's age level and maturity. Of course, we did our due diligence. As parents, we want the best for our children, but it's also good to let the child have a say in what happens with their bodies; they're the ones who have to go through all this. I'm so glad I allowed her to make that choice because she's 100% into it.

For this research opportunity, we have to go in once a month for infusion. During this trial stage, some people get the placebo and some get the real thing. They get their data from how the child reacts to it amongst other things. At this point, we don't know which one Saraya has been getting, but we think she's getting the real thing. It's a two-year trial. Once the last of the group goes through the treatment, then it'll be out there in the market. So far, so good! I think one of the reasons why she likes it is because they use the method of infusion and it's just once a month. She just goes, sits there, and they give her an infusion, and voilà, all done.

There are countless other research opportunities out there. From my understanding, gene cell therapy is when you take the cell from the patient and then it's altered. After that, they introduce it back into the patient's body. Gene cell therapy is being introduced for other kinds of diseases too. Bone marrow transplant is when they extract the bone marrow from the hip of someone who has the same cell or DNA as the patient and put it into the patient; the person has to be a perfect match, like a brother or sister with both of the same parents. Those are just layman's terms. Either way, in both cases (gene cell therapy and the bone marrow transplant), they have to go through chemotherapy. That was a no-no for Saraya because they explained everything that can happen during chemo: you can lose your hair, have breakouts, get a dry mouth, get sores, have skin problems and so many other side effects. On top of that, your body has to take in something foreign to it, and chances are that the patient's body could reject it. We've personally seen cases of that. Either way, with anything foreign that's introduced into the human body, there's a 50/50 chance that it'll work. Even with the infusion we do each month, after receiving treatment, she gets tired. That's the side effect she has, but it may look different for others because each patient is different.

There were three different options introduced to us: gene cell therapy, bone marrow transplant, and infusion. The latter is what she's doing now. The infusion helps to decrease the pain crises due to sickle cell, but it doesn't cure sickle cell.

PAIN-MANAGEMENT

The good thing about attending the Camp New Hope events is that they teach them how to manage their pain. They have them shift their mind away from the pain and focus on something else. This is a very good technique, as it allows you to project your mind to a happy place or a happy experience. That takes your mind away from the pain.

JOINING COMMUNITIES

After I left corporate America, I decided to get out of my comfort zone and join an online business network group to surround myself with like-minded entrepreneurs. One of my goals is to create a family business. Being a part of this group has opened up my mind to the endless possibilities available in entrepreneurship. We attend weekly zoom meetings which I look forward to.

That says a lot considering I used to hate meetings, because I felt that they were a waste of time. Since it's virtual, it makes it easy for me to attend. There's never a dull moment. I learn something new every day and gain many business tips.

What I've also discovered in this group is that there are no limitations. There are only limitations that I create for myself. If I put a barrier or limitation on my thinking, that's what I choose to succumb to. It's up to me. We're limitless in what we can accomplish, and whatever we set our minds to, we can accomplish.

Lately, I am more at ease. I think it's because our visits to the ER have somewhat lessened. I have more time on my hands to do the things I love to do, which includes creating financial wealth.

Advice from a caregiver.

(Taking care of yourself, mind, body, and soul)

Compassion is necessary. For yourself and your loved one & their experience.

Attitude is everything. Your perspective will shape the present moment.

Real love defines the time and energy spent on devoting yourself to your loved one.

Energy will help you to endure.

Gratitude helps tremendously.

Inspiration should be all around you.

Vitality. Don't ever take it for granted.

Embrace your life.

Resilience of the human spirit is your superpower.

I always strive to have a positive outlook on my situation. Please understand when I talk about being positive, I'm not saying I'm happy-go-lucky or even that there's a "happy" pill that you can take and everything will be perfect.

Yes, I do get depressed at times, and for the longest, I tried to hide it from my kids. I thought I was doing well with hiding it until one day, my daughter, Amaka, said, "why are you laying in bed? Are you depressed?"

I said, "Why are you saying that?"

She said, "Because depressed people do that."

I appreciate the awareness of millennials. I'm from the old school. We believe that you work through your stuff. It's okay to have someone to talk to, but I've always functioned by working through my difficulties. Through prayers and supplication, I take my request before God and He has never failed me. There's only so much a human being can do. I have close friends, but what do I expect them to do if I call them up announcing every time Saraya has a crisis? The only being that understands what I go through is God. Whether it's by bringing someone around or lightening the pressure on me, He always answers. It's not always in the way I think, but enough to be able to take the pressure off my mind that relieves stress and gives me peace.

Meditation also helps, because our thoughts are very powerful. I do go through rough patches, but I also give myself grace and remember that it's okay to worry or be angry sometimes, but to snap out of it. You can't sit in your funk for too long.

REFLECTIONS:

What role does different perspectives play in how you live your life? What would you recommend for other people who are going through crises and challenges to get out of a "victim" mentality?

____

____

____

____

____

____

____

____

____

CHANGE IS NORMAL

CHAPTER 7

Since my children are much older now, they tell me, "oh, I got this. I can take care of this." My thoughts proceeded like this: "If you feel you can take care of yourself, then you need to be out of my house. Because if you're in my house, you go by my rules."

They had just come back home from college for the holidays and were wanting to stay. In my mind, I had mapped out my life in such a way that I could shift my focus from all of them to just Saraya and then hopefully myself.

I gave them a timeline to get their acts together and figure out what they wanted to do. This timeframe was 6 months, to be exact. It was during COVID-19 time, and in my mind, I just felt they were taking their sweet time to make their move. They hated when I would tell them what to do, but of course, as parents, that's what we do. I would pick at little things to make it uncomfortable for them to continue living in my house. When I'd raise my voice at them and snap at them, they'd tell me to chill and relax. At this stage, they want their privacy, so I make it difficult for them to be private in my house.

In my head, I was thinking, "Okay, you are young adults now, so you've gotta get busy." They were making some headway in their own way, but I guess since I had already painted the picture in my head that I had been a single parent for many years and after Saraya went off to college, I'd mapped out that I would focus on my wellbeing and mindset. So suddenly when I saw them trying to ease their way back into the home, I'm like, "ah, that's not happening. No, no." This is why I gave them a timeframe. I understand that things do happen, so I'm here for my kids, but they are still expected to get it together.

I LOVE MY THINGS

They know I love my things. If you take something, put it back where you found it. It's that simple. I'm not saying not to touch it. I'd prefer they ask for permission, but at the least, I expect them to make sure it's back where they found it. If that thing is moved elsewhere and I'm looking for it, I have a problem with that. That's a big thing in my household. Sometimes, I just don't understand why if they know what I like and are aware of what I've taught them, why they won't comply. It's a teachable moment, because now when they go out into the real world and do that same thing to someone else, it's a negative reflection of the family they came from.

That's just how I was raised. The funny thing is that they are just so well-behaved out there in the real world, but when they're home, they give me unsettling moments. I was raised on tough love, and so

I am passing that down to them. When they get out of line, I nip it in the bud. I just correct them immediately. I don't like to let it sit and simmer; I just act on it. To this day I continue that. They don't like it but are used to it.

First off, when they left for college and during the holidays, they gave me the impression that they were okay. They said they found their place and that they were leaving. You know how kids are though. When you say something to them and they want to talk back, then they're like, "oh, I'm gonna get my own place." Fine. Yeah. It's like, "there's the door." I told them that wouldn't be a problem, and in fact, it'd be perfect for me. They tried to make me feel guilty but I knew that it was time for me to focus on myself in addition to Saraya's health.

Yakoub and Amaka are very good at keeping up with Saraya because they check in on her, almost every other day. When they were leaving for college, she was the one who felt their absence because they were all quite close to each other. She was very saddened by it, but I told her, "well, they're going off to college, so it's natural for them to be away from the house."

She's at a point where she enjoys her solitude. Once in a while, they stop by for a visit but she knows they're always a phone call away. It's no longer a problem. As much as I wanted them to leave the home, as a mother, you tend to kind of worry for your kids to some extent, no matter what age they are. That's where prayer comes in, because I was stressing myself. I just went to God in prayer and said, "you know what? If I say I have committed these kids into your care, then I have to trust that you're taking care of them and have taken this burden from me." That has worked for me. Now, they always feel as if I'm a phone call away. "Mommy, can you help with this?" "Mom? Can you do that?" I'm getting to the point where I'm saying "no" more often than not. I think they hear it in my voice. Sometimes when they call, I'm automatically like, "WHAT?!" I love them so much though.

MIDLIFE CRISIS THOUGHT MODE

I guess what it comes down to is that I wanted to finally experience a life of my own. I'm getting close to what I like to call semi-retirement, and the 2.5 years left for Saraya in high school will go by really fast. I knew I had to figure myself out. As caregivers and also single moms, there's a tendency to give your whole life to your kids; you do everything for them. You don't want to get to a point when they're all grown and have left the house that you feel empty inside. We go through a midlife crisis. When this happens, we ask ourselves, "What's gonna happen now?" because we've placed so much of our identity into being just a parent. For me, I decided that I need to start now and just figure out what it is I want to do.

So, why do I need a life of my own? Women sometimes get in their feelings. It's just the cycle of life and how we are wired. I'm not going to leave the men out here though. I imagine this also happens in two-parent homes and single-father homes. You get to a point where you've done your due diligence with your kids, and you feel you want to do something for yourself. Naturally, the kids will come back every so often, but you get the nerve to say, "you know what? I've done enough for you. Now, I need to take care of myself."

My next phase includes me figuring it out little by little as I go on. This book is a stepping stone towards that. It's a release to talk about my experiences and what I've been through. I know and believe there are others out there who are going through the same and who have gone through worse than I've gone through, and who are being impacted positively by reading this book. I know the possibilities are endless, and I plan to do all that I love to do.

REFLECTIONS:

What major changes have you experienced in your life? In what ways would you like to honor yourself moving forward?

GROWTH IS SOMETIMES INEVITABLE

CHAPTER 8

SHE SPROUTED OVERNIGHT, IT SEEMS

When Saraya came to me and said she wanted to move to Seattle. I asked her why and she said she just feels like it. I quickly went to research the city. And I said, "you know, it rains there a lot?"

She said, "yeah, I love the rain."

She loves the weather. I said, okay. In my mind, I'd imagine it to be much like California. As I continued my research, I told her, "Okay, well maybe we could take a road trip there. Let's see what it looks like."

We have yet to do that. She said she wanted the whole family to go. She wanted her siblings to go and they didn't have time, but that's still something on our bucket list. We plan on going out there to explore because she was saying she would like to go to college there. She came up with Seattle of all places. Nothing wrong with that. I'll cross that mental hurdle when the time comes. (wink)

GRANDMOTHER

I was blessed with a grandson during COVID-19. He's boisterous and has so much energy. He keeps us on our feet. I call him my little man and he's very smart. Like both his parents.

THE PROBLEM WITH STIGMA

Saraya and all those individuals battling this sickle cell disease are warriors, as we like to call them. Because they're codependent on their medication due to the pain crisis, they have to battle against the stigma of society looking at them in a certain way. They're constantly being stigmatized. First, most people don't understand their circumstances and conditions. With the opioid crisis going on, it just makes their situation worse. Depending on their age, they are judged for their need for pain medication. As a child, it's accepted because you are going to walk into the hospital accompanied by your caregiver, but I think when they become adults, they don't get much support.

Children with SCD may face social stigma and discrimination due to the disease. Caregivers need to advocate for their child's rights and ensure that they receive fair treatment and access to education, employment, and healthcare.

I've heard of cases where some of these kids go off to college and they have a crisis, but when they go into the hospital, they are refused the proper treatment. This is not just something that only happens here in the states, but in other countries too. In addition to the students, it happens with older adults where the medical staff may not understand the disease; they tend to doubt the patients. This social stigma is what sickle cell warriors are up against.

As the parent of a young adult, I know that now I can control what anyone will say to my kid, but can you imagine if they're on their own?! That's something I constantly think about and I'm sure other caregivers think about it as well. This doesn't make it easy, but I have to trust that Saraya will do well on her own.

Children in this predicament should learn self-care early on to be able to take care of themselves because there are so many things we need to be able to do for ourselves naturally. Some of those things include making sure they're well hydrated, knowing their conditions throughout the day, and being aware of what can trigger them. Sometimes it can be difficult to know what triggers the pain crisis, but it's best to try to take precautions. It could be anything, especially stress. There are some ways you can control stress, but sometimes it just comes upon you without notice. I try to encourage my daughter to pay attention to her triggers; she knows her body better than anyone else. She can control what she ingests, how she takes care of herself, take proper nutrition to eat well, try her best to live a stress-free life, and most importantly, be able to speak up for herself. Sickle cell warriors have to advocate their condition. I'm beginning to see more and more sickle cell patients speaking up and bringing awareness to this disease.

MUSIC IS IMPORTANT

Yakoub is a self-taught musician. He taught Saraya to play the guitar. She developed a good ear for music. And during COVID-19 she was able to focus on creating and writing songs.

To be honest, when I read stories online from other people who are going through the same thing, I see that they say they're successful. Some doctors and professionals have sickle cell. The ones in Saraya's age group that I meet at the hospital have concerns. These youths in other countries don't want to be put in certain groups and viewed as incompetent; they want to thrive and expect to be treated as such. From my standpoint as a caregiver, I do have concerns, especially since she is my last born. I need to be careful about that though. As a parent, when you think less of what your child can do, they will surprise you. As she's growing, she has a certain strength and determination about herself and is committed to doing what she wants to do, and I respect her for that. I've learned to let her thrive and make her path. With that, I let her know that no matter what

she's going through, I'm always here. That's the conversation we've been having lately.

Amaka seems to think I'm like a helicopter parent. I know Saraya is getting to a point where she will
be done with high school and will have to choose
what she wants to do. Amaka thinks I'm very protective of Saraya because of her sickness, but she
doesn't know every single thing I've had to go
through.

Yes, I still worry even though I know that worry-
ing won't change anything. For now, we focus on
making sure she stays healthy and pain-free. For
me, it's more so stressful when she's stressed out,
so the goal is to minimize stress as much as possible.

REFLECTIONS:

What conversations do you have with your loved one about their dreams or how they feel? How do you balance helping and believing in them with helping and believing in yourself?

____

____

____

____

____

____

____

____

____

EPILOGUE

Caregivers need to educate themselves about SCD and how to manage the disease. There are several research opportunities regarding SCD pain crises. When parents go to the hospital, their goal should be to ask the hard questions and even those that may seem small. I kept asking questions about research opportunities when Saraya was younger. Most times, they would tell me, "oh, they closed this opportunity," or "Oh, she's too young for that." Meanwhile, other states like New York, Boston, California, and Ohio, had research programs taking place. Know your options; there may be an opportunity where you may have to travel out of state.

I kept asking and finally, something opened up here in Georgia. When you fill out your medical paperwork, they often ask, "if there are any research opportunities, will you be interested?" I always said, "Yes!" I think that's something parents should do. There's a tendency within our community not to want to put your children through research because of negative experiments and things that have happened in the past, but someone has to start somewhere. The advancements and treatments we now enjoy are the result of someone else's experience and now we can benefit from it. You can also look at it as paying it forward.

By getting help for my daughter, I feel I'm helping other kids out there too, just as other kids have helped us by participating in the program even before her. There's also a global sense of connection felt by being a part of that group because it's not just here in the states but a worldwide group. I believe we're doing something for the greater good. The beauty of it is that it's free. Of course, research is always free.

We may sometimes forget to take care of ourselves. I have to constantly remind myself that I can't give of myself if I have nothing within me to give. Oftentimes, we put ourselves on the back burner; I'm not just talking about our generation, but I'm sure our parents as well. We do so much and get to a point where we can go no further. It doesn't make sense. Our loved ones want us to always be around for as long as we can, but to lead healthy lives. It's extremely important as caregivers to practice self-care; we need to take care of our mindset.

To take care of myself, I started doing meditation. I also pray and read a lot. I could read anything and everything. I just love to read to expand my knowledge. Lately, I've been interested in mental health. (chuckles) How befitting, because that's something that's been a big issue with COVID-19. A lot of people are losing their minds. People are tired.

And for a good reason. If you've been cooped up for a long time, suddenly you are wondering what's the essence of life. That also comes with age; you get to a point where you're like, "what have I done?" It's like, your life has passed you by, and there's just so much out there to be done. So I love to read and research. And now, I guess you can add writing. (smiles)

SARAYA

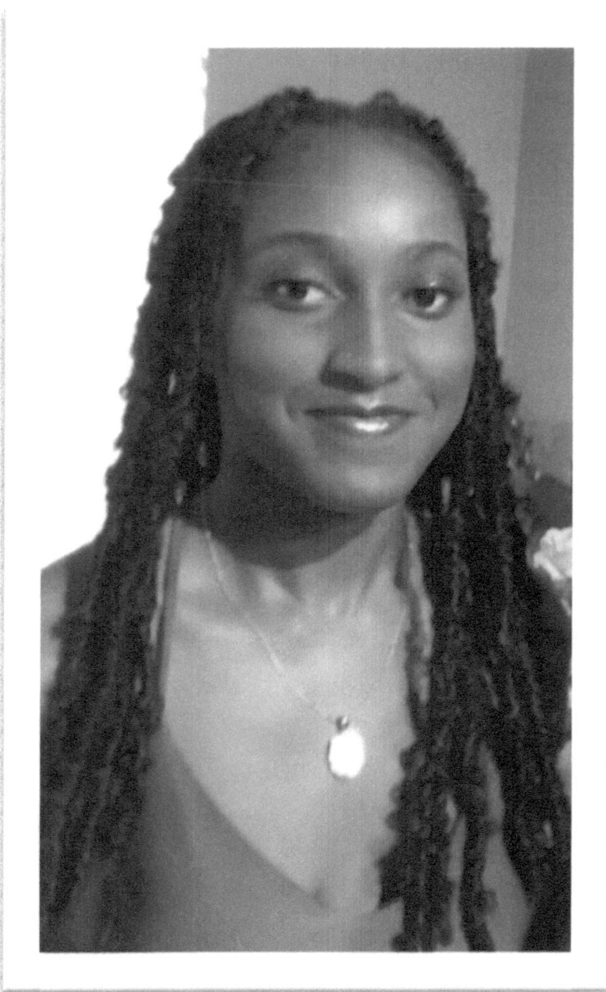

FEAR

What am I afraid of…
Losing you to this 'beast'
ANGER
No not angry
FRUSTRATION is what I feel
Why?
Because it takes me away from the usual
COMPASSION
I see you battling with the pain
I feel how much you try so hard
And yet I'm helpless
Because I can't shield you
I can only watch as you battle this beast
All I have is God's promise
To see you through these crises
And His promise to
"preserve your going out
And your coming in this time
forth and forevermore"

ACKNOWLEDGEMENTS

I am **eternally** grateful to God for the experience of motherhood and also the opportunity. As I mentioned in the book, I lived a 'sheltered' life prior to going through this life-altering experience. Before now, I didn't have to be in the hospital or ER ever so often. So while this may be unpleasant, for the most part, it has kept me grounded and grateful for each day I and my loved ones get to experience life and good health…. Because despite everything I have been given the strength and fortitude to deal with this curveball.

Also, I'm grateful to my children Yakoub, Amaka, and Saraya for their encouragement and support. Without you, there wouldn't be a need to write this story. You push me to see what I can't seem to see in myself. You give me a reason to get up each day even when I honestly don't feel like it. Your belief that I had something valuable to share has kept me going even through my self-doubt and uncertainty.

I'm so grateful to Andrea for taking a chance on me and helping to make this book come to fruition.

Special thanks to the caring doctors, nurses, and caregivers at Children's Healthcare of Atlanta at

Scottish Rite who have graciously cared for my daughter as well as other children over the years.

Equally important to mention are the different foundations that give their time and effort by bringing food and care products to the families and patients while on admission; we truly appreciate your efforts.

To Daryl 'Bey', your silent strength and support, I will always hold dear to my heart.

I'm also very thankful to my family and friends for their thoughts and prayers on Saraya's health. It does take a village.

ABOUT THE AUTHOR

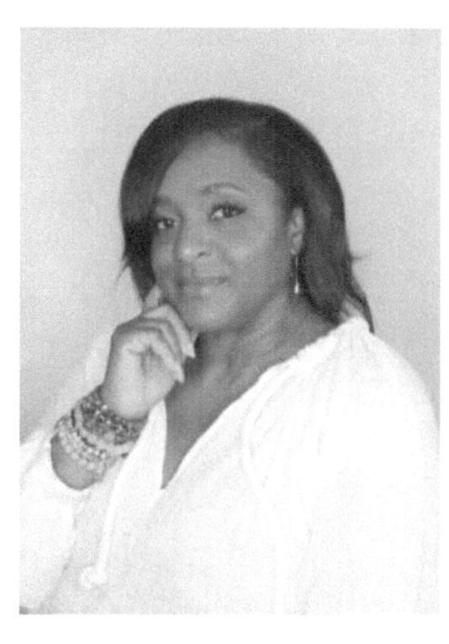

Pippa Maha was born in Lagos, Nigeria to parents, Philip and Victoria Maha. While in Nigeria, she earned her diploma in TV Production and moved to Brazil as a young adult, where she earned her first degree in International Relations. Pippa grew up surrounded by different cultures and loves to cook, read, and critique movies, art, and music. She later relocated to the United States and earned her MBA in Global Business, while working in the Property and Casualty Insurance industry for two decades. Her mission is to motivate others who are going through life changes and traumatic experiences to find a way to live an elevated life by sharing her experience through public speaking, mentorship, and her literary works. She believes that "everything we go through in life prepares us for our next sequence in life" and that we all have a "universal connection" that we get glimpses of through our food, culture, music, and self-expression. Pippa enjoys spending time with her children, grandson, and her dog, Osha, affectionately known as Chickboo.

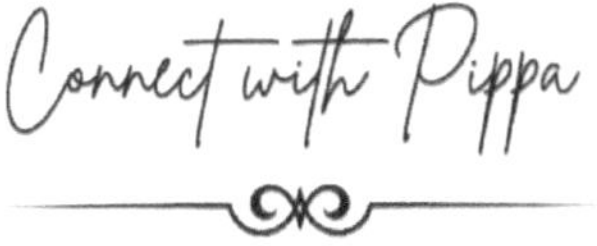

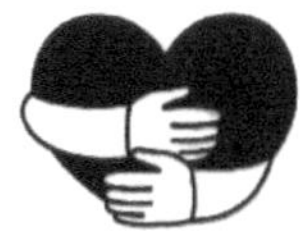

To learn more about Pippa and her support group for caregivers, email support@abbashirleywellness.com

Connect with Pippa Maha by scanning the code below.
- Please leave a review for *I'm Not Your Superwoman.*
- Inquire about her speaking services for your next event or organization meeting.
- Join her support group for caregivers.

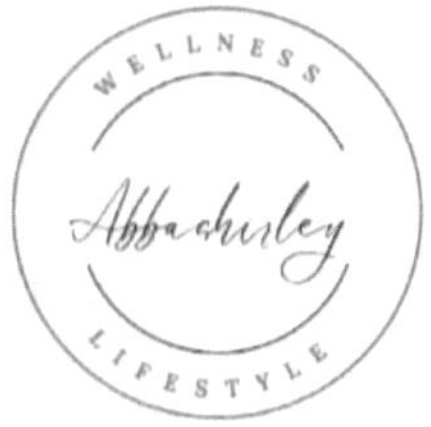

PIPPA'S FAVORITE JUICE RECIPES

Iron-clad Juice

1 beet

1 apple

A knob of ginger

Green Goddess Juice

3 stalks of celery

1 green apple

A knob of ginger

1 lemon

Clear Skin Juice

2 carrots

1 orange

A knob of ginger

Do you have a desire to write your own book? Schedule a discovery call with Andrea "Kitten" Perry to get the help you need with writing your book, & become one of our next authors.
Go to www.beautifulbookgoddess.com

Want to be included in the next Yonitry book, but not sure if you have what it takes to write heartfelt, thought-provoking poetry? Sign up for the next WRITE LIKE YONI workshop by scanning this code and clicking on the option, "Write Like Yoni." Take advantage of this opportunity to join the sisterhood.

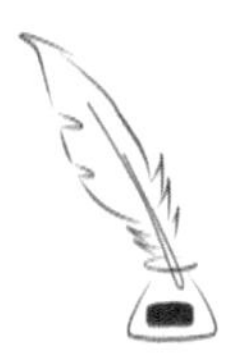

Need book publishing services?
Contact us at
publishing@ismetfreepress.com
or visit www.ismetfreepress.com
to learn how we can assist you in birthing your nonfiction masterpiece.

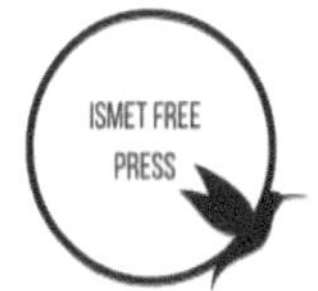

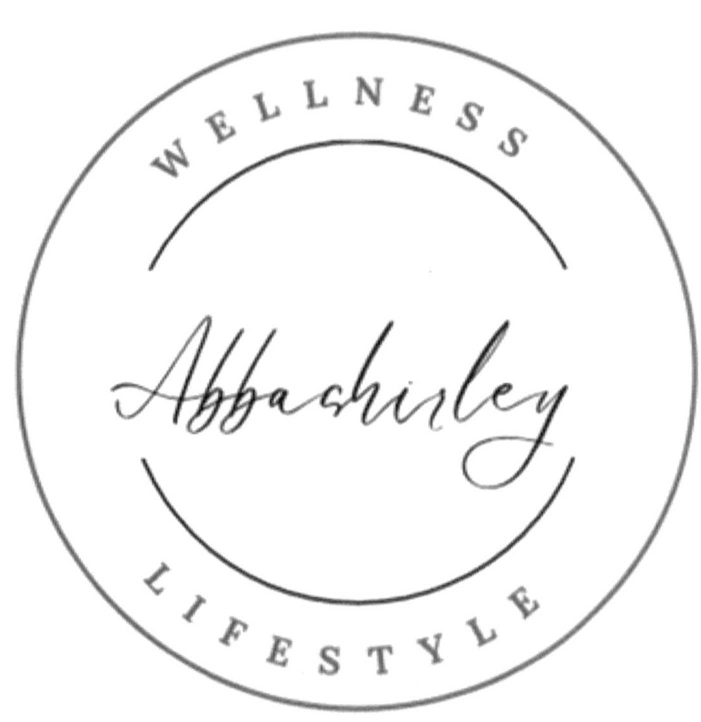

WELLNESS
Abbashirley
LIFESTYLE